# HEALTHY EATING COOKBOOK FOR MEN ABOVE 60

## Easy nutritional guide for seniors to stay strong, prevent sickness as they continue to age

By

AUTHUR QUINN

# Copyright

Copyright © 2024 [Your Name or Your Publishing Entity]

# TABLE OF CONT

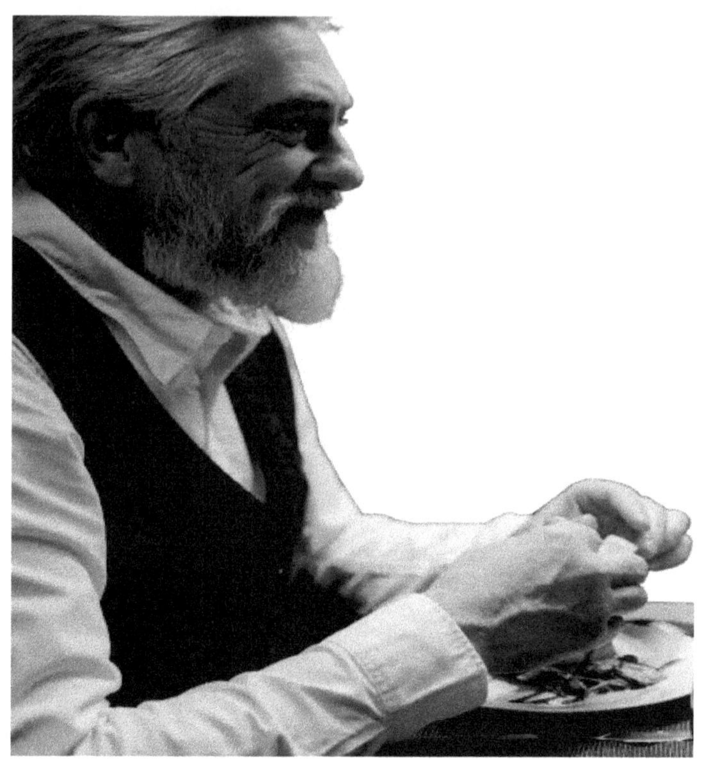

# Introduction

In a world where time seems to quicken its pace, men above 60 find themselves at a crucial juncture, where the choices they make profoundly impact their well-being. Embracing a lifestyle centered around healthy eating becomes more than a mere choice; it transforms into a beacon guiding them towards a vibrant and fulfilling life.

Meet Robert, a spirited 63-year-old who decided to embark on a journey of rejuvenation through mindful nutrition. His story mirrors the experiences of countless men navigating the challenges of aging. As he delved into the realm of healthy eating, Robert discovered that it wasn't about restrictive diets but rather a harmonious balance of nutrients tailored to his changing needs.

The narrative unfolds in his kitchen, where vibrant fruits, vegetables, and whole grains take center stage. Gone are the days of processed convenience; instead, Robert embraces homemade meals crafted with care. His journey isn't just about shedding unhealthy habits; it's a celebration of savoring nutrient-rich foods that nourish his body and mind.

In this exploration of the importance of eating well after 60, we encounter not just Robert but a community of men who have embraced this transformative shift. Their stories echo the sentiment that healthy eating isn't a sacrifice but a gift—one that bestows increased energy, enhanced cognitive function, and resilience against the trials of aging.

As we delve into the **Healthy Eating Cookbook for men above 60**, we unravel the science behind it all. From essential vitamins and minerals to the role of hydration, this narrative serves as a compass for those seeking to make informed choices about their diet. Join us on a journey where forks become tools of empowerment, and every bite is a step towards a healthier, more vibrant future.

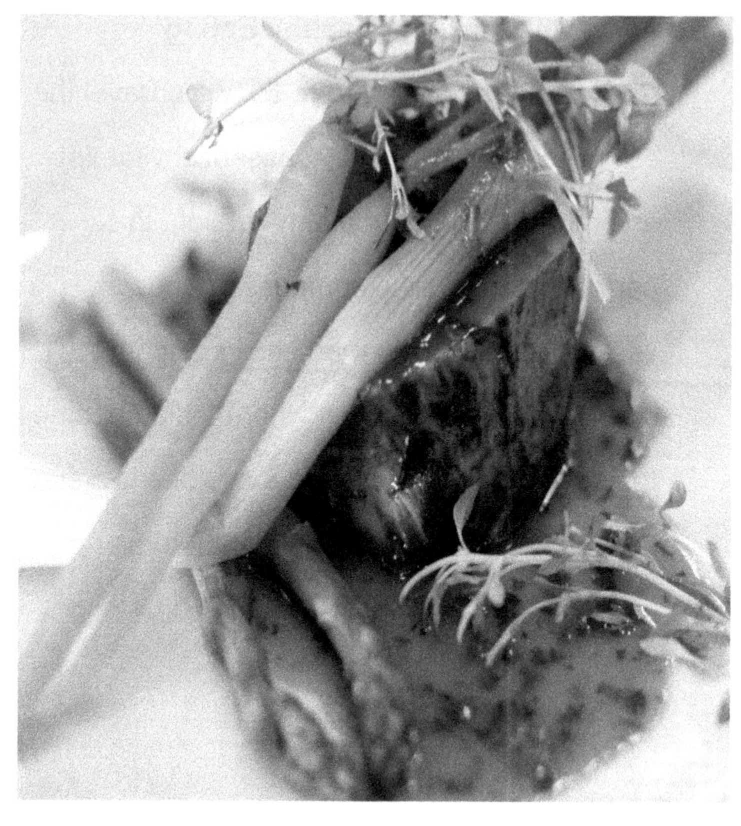

# Chapter one

## What eating healthy is and what it is not:

Eating healthy involves consuming a well-balanced diet rich in nutrients, including fruits, vegetables, whole grains, lean proteins, and healthy fats. It prioritizes moderation, variety, and portion control to support overall well-being.

On the contrary, unhealthy eating often involves excessive intake of processed foods, sugary snacks, and high-fat, high-calorie meals. It may lack essential nutrients, leading to imbalances and potential health issues. Eating healthy is not about extreme diets or

deprivation but rather making sustainable
choices for long-term health.

# Benefits of eating healthy for seniors above 60:

Eating healthy is crucial for seniors above 60
as it provides numerous benefits that
contribute to overall well-being and quality of
life. Here are some extensive reasons why
maintaining a nutritious diet is particularly
important for older adults:

1. **Nutrient Adequacy**: Seniors have
   specific nutritional needs, and a
   balanced diet ensures they receive an
   adequate intake of essential nutrients
   such as vitamins, minerals, protein, and

fiber. This helps in maintaining optimal bodily functions and supports the immune system.

2. **Bone Health**: Calcium and vitamin D are vital for maintaining bone health, reducing the risk of osteoporosis and fractures, common concerns for seniors. A diet rich in dairy products, leafy greens, and fortified foods can contribute to bone strength.

3. **Heart Health**: A heart-healthy diet, low in saturated fats and cholesterol, can help manage blood pressure and cholesterol levels. This reduces the risk of cardiovascular diseases, which become more prevalent in older age.

4. **Weight Management**: Maintaining a healthy weight is crucial for seniors to prevent issues such as obesity and

associated conditions like diabetes. A nutrient-dense diet, combined with regular physical activity, supports weight management.

5. **Cognitive Function**: Certain nutrients, such as omega-3 fatty acids and antioxidants found in fish, fruits, and vegetables, have been linked to improved cognitive function. A diet rich in these elements may help reduce the risk of cognitive decline in older adults.

6. **Digestive Health**: Fiber-rich foods aid in digestion and help prevent constipation, a common issue among seniors. Whole grains, fruits, and vegetables contribute to a healthy digestive system.

7. **Hydration**: Staying adequately hydrated is crucial for seniors, as dehydration can lead to various health complications.

Drinking enough water supports proper bodily functions, including kidney function and temperature regulation.

8. **Reduced Inflammation**: Chronic inflammation is associated with many age-related diseases. Antioxidant-rich foods, such as berries and leafy greens, can help combat inflammation, promoting better health in seniors.

9. **Improved Energy Levels**: A balanced diet provides the necessary energy for daily activities. Seniors who consume nutrient-rich meals are likely to experience improved energy levels, supporting an active lifestyle.

10. **Mood and Mental Health:** Nutrient-rich foods contribute to the production of neurotransmitters that affect mood. A healthy diet can positively influence

mental well-being, reducing the risk of
depression and anxiety in seniors.

11. **Enhanced Immune Function**:
Adequate nutrition supports a robust
immune system, which becomes
increasingly important as the body's
defenses naturally weaken with age.
Vitamins and minerals from fruits,
vegetables, and lean proteins contribute
to immune health.

12. **Disease Prevention**: A nutritious diet
plays a key role in preventing various
chronic diseases, including diabetes,
hypertension, and certain types of
cancer, which seniors are more
susceptible to.

In summary, eating a healthy, well-balanced
diet is essential for seniors above 60 to

promote physical health, mental well-being, and longevity. It serves as a foundation for overall wellness, helping them enjoy an active and fulfilling life in their golden year

## Typical health issues that males above 60 face;

Men over 60 commonly face a range of health issues, often influenced by factors such as genetics, lifestyle, and overall health history. Some prevalent health concerns in this demographic include:

1. **Cardiovascular Diseases**: As men age, the risk of heart diseases, including coronary artery disease, heart failure,

and hypertension, increases. Regular check-ups, a heart-healthy diet, and exercise are crucial for cardiovascular health.

2. **Prostate Issues**: Enlargement of the prostate, known as benign prostatic hyperplasia (BPH), is common among older men and can lead to urinary problems. Prostate cancer risk also rises with age, necessitating regular screenings.

3. **Osteoporosis**: While often associated with women, men are also susceptible to bone density loss. Osteoporosis increases the risk of fractures, and maintaining a diet rich in calcium and vitamin D, along with weight-bearing exercises, helps mitigate this risk.

4.  **Diabetes**: The prevalence of diabetes tends to rise with age. Regular blood sugar monitoring, a healthy diet, and exercise play vital roles in managing diabetes and preventing complications.

5.  **Vision and Hearing Loss**: Aging often brings about changes in vision and hearing. Regular eye and ear check-ups are essential for early detection and management of issues such as cataracts, glaucoma, and hearing loss.

6.  **Arthritis and Joint Problems**: Conditions like osteoarthritis become more common with age, leading to joint pain and reduced mobility. Exercise, weight management, and joint-friendly activities can help alleviate symptoms.

7.  **Neurological Conditions**: Cognitive decline, Alzheimer's disease, and other

forms of dementia become more prevalent in older age. Mental stimulation, a healthy diet, and social engagement may contribute to maintaining cognitive function.

8. **Respiratory Issues:** Chronic obstructive pulmonary disease (COPD) and other respiratory problems become more common as men age. Smoking cessation, regular exercise, and proper medical management are crucial for lung health.

9. **Skin Conditions**: Skin becomes more susceptible to various issues, including dryness, age spots, and skin cancer. Regular dermatological check-ups, sun protection, and a skincare routine help address these concerns.

10. **Weight Management and Metabolic Changes:** Aging often leads to a decrease in metabolism and muscle mass, making weight management challenging. A balanced diet and regular physical activity are essential for maintaining a healthy weight.

Regular health check-ups, preventive measures, and a healthy lifestyle can significantly contribute to maintaining overall well-being for men over 60. It's important for individuals in this age group to work closely with healthcare professionals to address specific health concerns and develop personalized care plans.

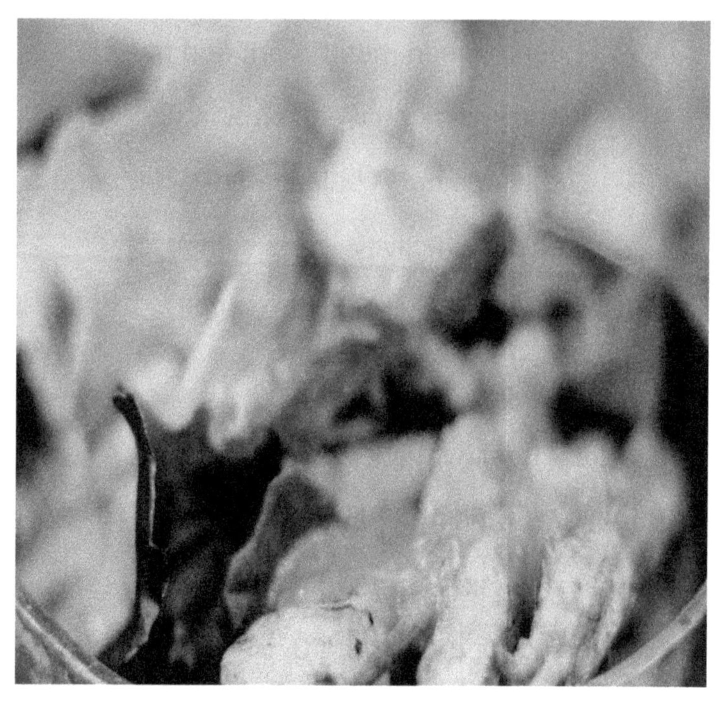

# CHAPTER TWO

## Nutritional needs for men above 60;

Nutritional needs for men above 60 are crucial for maintaining overall health and well-being. As individuals age, their bodies undergo various changes, including alterations in metabolism, bone density, muscle mass, and hormonal balance. Proper nutrition becomes increasingly important to support these changes and reduce the risk of age-related health issues. Here's an overview of key nutritional considerations for men in this age group:

1. **Protein Intake:**
    - Adequate protein intake is essential for maintaining muscle mass, strength, and overall body function.

- Include lean protein sources such as poultry, fish, eggs, dairy, legumes, and plant-based proteins in the diet.

2. **Calcium and Vitamin D:**
   - Bone health becomes a significant concern as men age. Calcium and vitamin D are crucial for maintaining strong bones and preventing osteoporosis.
   - Dairy products, leafy green vegetables, fortified foods, and sunlight exposure are good sources.

3. **Fiber-Rich Foods:**
   - A diet high in fiber helps support digestive health, regulate blood sugar levels, and manage weight.
   - Incorporate whole grains, fruits, vegetables, and legumes to ensure an ample fiber intake.

4. **Heart-Healthy Fats:**
   - Opt for healthy fats like omega-3 fatty acids, found in fish, flaxseeds, and walnuts, to support cardiovascular health.
   - Limit saturated and trans fats by reducing processed and fried foods.

5. **Hydration**:
   - Staying hydrated is essential for maintaining overall health, supporting organ function, and preventing dehydration-related issues.
   - Try to consume 8 glasses of water or more each day, and think about including foods high in water content, such as fruits and vegetables.
6. **Antioxidant-Rich Foods**:
   - Antioxidants help combat oxidative stress and inflammation, which can contribute to age-related diseases.
   - Include colorful fruits and vegetables, nuts, seeds, and green tea in the diet.
7. **Vitamins and Minerals:**
   - Ensure a well-balanced intake of vitamins and minerals by consuming a variety of foods.
   - Consider supplementation if there are deficiencies, but consult with a healthcare professional before doing so.
8. **Portion Control:**

- Metabolism tends to slow down with age, making portion control crucial for maintaining a healthy weight.
  - Pay attention to portion sizes and listen to hunger cues to prevent overeating.

9. **Limit Sodium Intake:**
   - Limit your sodium consumption to help control blood pressure and promote heart health.
   - Choose fresh, whole foods over processed and packaged items, and use herbs and spices for flavoring.

10. **Regular Physical Activity**:
    - Nutrition goes hand in hand with physical activity. Regular exercise helps maintain muscle mass, bone density, and overall health.
    - Engage in a mix of cardiovascular, strength, and flexibility exercises, tailored to individual cap

# Breakfast delight for men above 60;

A wholesome breakfast is crucial for men above 60, providing essential nutrients to support overall health and well-being. Incorporating a balanced mix of proteins, carbohydrates, fiber, and vitamins is key. Consider a combination of the following elements to create a delightful and nourishing breakfast:

**Protein Power**::Include protein-rich foods like eggs, lean meats, or Greek yogurt. These promote muscle health, aid in tissue repair, and provide a sense of fullness.

**Fiber-Filled** Grains::Opt for whole grains like oatmeal, whole wheat bread, or bran cereals. These not only offer sustained energy but also support digestive health and help manage cholesterol levels.

**Healthy Fats**:Incorporate sources of healthy fats such as avocados, nuts, and seeds. These contribute to heart health and help absorb fat-soluble vitamins.

**Colorful Fruits**:;Include a variety of fruits for their vitamins, antioxidants, and natural sweetness. Bananas, citrus fruits, and berries are great options.

**Calcium Boosters**:Dairy or dairy alternatives can provide essential calcium for bone health. Consider low-fat milk, fortified plant-based milks, or yogurt.

**Hydration is Key**:Start the day with a glass of water to rehydrate after a night's sleep. Herbal teas or 100% fruit juices can also be good options.

**Mindful Portions**:Pay attention to portion sizes to avoid overeating. A well-balanced breakfast should provide enough energy without causing discomfort.

**Special Considerations**:If there are specific health concerns, consult with a healthcare professional or nutritionist to tailor the breakfast to individual needs. For example, those with diabetes might focus on managing carbohydrate intake.

**Variety is the Spice of Life**:Rotate breakfast options to keep things interesting and ensure a diverse range of nutrients. This could include switching between different grains, proteins, and fruits.

**Preparation Techniques**:Choose healthy cooking methods such as steaming, boiling, or grilling to preserve nutritional content. Limit the use of added sugars and excessive salt.

Remember, a breakfast tailored to the nutritional needs of men above 60 can contribute to improved energy levels, cognitive function, and overall health. It's a good idea to personalize these suggestions based on personal preferences and dietary restrictions

# Wholesome Lunches;

A wholesome lunch for men above 60 should focus on a balanced combination of nutrients to support their overall health and well-being. Consider including lean proteins, whole grains, fruits, vegetables, and healthy fats in their meals. Some ideas for a nutritious lunch include:

1. **Protein-rich options:**
    - Grilled chicken or turkey breast: Provides essential amino acids and is low in saturated fat.
    - Fish (such as salmon or tuna): Rich in omega-3 fatty acids, beneficial for heart health.

- Legumes (beans, lentils): Excellent plant-based protein sources with fiber and vitamins.

2. **Whole grains:**

   - Brown rice: A good source of fiber, vitamins, and minerals.
   - Quinoa: Packed with protein, fiber, and various nutrients.
   - Whole-grain bread or pasta: Provides sustained energy and essential nutrients.

3. **Vegetables**:

   - Dark leafy greens (spinach, kale): High in vitamins, minerals, and antioxidants.
   - Colorful vegetables (bell peppers, carrots): Provide a range of nutrients and add flavor.

4. **Healthy fats:**

- Avocado: Offers
      monounsaturated fats and
      various vitamins.
    - Olive oil: Use for cooking or in
      dressings for its heart-healthy
      benefits.

5. **Dairy or dairy alternatives**:
    - Greek yogurt or low-fat yogurt:
      Rich in protein and calcium for
      bone health.
    - Almond or soy milk: Suitable
      alternatives for those with lactose
      intolerance.

6. **Fruits**:
    - Berries (blueberries,
      strawberries): Packed with
      antioxidants and vitamins.
    - Apple or pear: Good sources of
      fiber and natural sweetness.

7.  **Hydration**:

   - Water: Ensure proper hydration throughout the day for overall health.
   - Herbal teas: Provide additional hydration with potential health benefits.

8.  **Portion control**:

   - Pay attention to portion sizes to maintain a healthy weight and prevent overeating.

9.  **Limit processed foods:**

   - Minimize the intake of processed and high-sodium foods to support heart health.

10. **Customization**:

   - Consider any dietary restrictions or preferences, and adjust the meal accordingly.

Remember to consult with a healthcare professional or a registered dietitian to create a personalized meal plan based on individual health needs and preferences.

**Wholesome Lunch Options for Men Above 60 – Mediterranean Style:**

Embracing a Mediterranean-inspired lunch can offer numerous health benefits for men above 60. This diet is renowned for promoting heart health and overall well-being. Consider these elements for a wholesome Mediterranean lunch:

**Lean Proteins**:Grilled fish (like Mediterranean favorites such as sardines or mackerel): Rich in omega-3 fatty acids for cardiovascular health.

Skinless poultry (chicken or turkey): A lean source of protein.

**Whole Grains:**Couscous or bulgur: Nutrient-dense whole grains that provide fiber and essential minerals.

Whole-grain pita bread: A delightful addition for fiber and sustained energy.

**Healthy Fats:**Olive oil: A staple in Mediterranean cuisine, offering monounsaturated fats with anti-inflammatory properties.

**Nuts and seeds (almonds, walnuts, flaxseeds):** Provide additional healthy fats and a crunchy texture.

**Abundance of Vegetables:**Tomatoes, cucumbers, and bell peppers: Rich in

**antioxidants and vitamins.**Leafy greens (arugula, spinach): Enhance nutritional content and flavor.

**Herbs and Spices**:Basil, oregano, and rosemary: Boost flavor without the need for excessive salt.

**Garlic**: Known for its potential health benefits, including cardiovascular support.

**Dairy or Dairy Alternatives:**Feta or goat cheese: Adds a creamy texture and a unique taste.

**Greek yogurt**: High in protein and beneficial probiotics.

**Colorful Fruits:**Berries, figs, or citrus fruits: Rich in vitamins, antioxidants, and natural sweetness.

**Hydration**:Water infused with citrus slices or a splash of mint for refreshing hydration.

**Red wine (in moderation):** Offers potential heart health benefits.

**Portion Control and Mindful Eating**:Savor each bite, focusing on the flavors and textures.

For better digestion, choose smaller, more frequent meals.

**Social Aspects**:Consider sharing meals with family or friends, fostering a positive and enjoyable dining experience.

## Balanced and Nourishing Lunches for Men Above 60 – Asian Fusion:

Crafting a lunch inspired by Asian flavors can provide a balance of tastes and nutrients for men above 60. Incorporate the following elements for a wholesome and culturally diverse meal:

1. **Lean Proteins:**
   - Grilled or stir-fried tofu: A plant-based protein source.
   - Chicken or shrimp: Rich in protein with a variety of cooking options.

2. **Whole Grains**:
   - Brown rice or quinoa: Fiber-rich choices offering sustained energy.

- Soba or udon noodles: Japanese
    noodles providing a unique twist.

3. **Healthy Fats:**

   - Sesame oil: Adds a distinct flavor
     and provides healthy fats.

   - Avocado: Offers
     monounsaturated fats for heart
     health.

4. **Abundance of Vegetables:**

   - Stir-fried broccoli, bok choy, and
     bell peppers: Packed with
     vitamins and antioxidants.

   - Mushrooms: A nutritious addition
     with a savory umami flavor.

5. **Herbs and Spices**:

   - Ginger and garlic: Infuse depth of
     flavor with potential health
     benefits.

- Turmeric: Known for its anti-inflammatory properties.

6. **Dairy or Dairy Alternatives:**

   - Incorporate coconut milk in curries for a creamy texture.
   - Tofu as a dairy-free protein alternative.

7. **Colorful Fruits:**

   - Mango or pineapple: Sweet and refreshing additions.
   - Citrus fruits: Provide a burst of vitamin C.

8. **Tea Options:**

   - Green tea or herbal teas: Offer hydration with potential health benefits.
   - Avoid excessive sugary drinks for optimal health.

9.  **Portion Control and Balanced Composition:**
    - Create a well-balanced plate with a mix of proteins, grains, and vegetables.
    - Control portion sizes to support overall health.

10. **Culinary Exploration**:
    - Experiment with different Asian cuisines, exploring the diverse array of flavors and ingredients.
    - Embrace the social aspect of dining, sharing meals with loved ones.

# A nourishing dinner for men above 60;

This should focus on providing essential nutrients to support overall health and address potential age-related concerns. Here's a comprehensive guide:

## Protein Sources:

**Grilled Chicken Breast:**Opt for lean proteins like grilled chicken breast, which provides essential amino acids for muscle maintenance.

**Lentils or Beans:**Include legumes like lentils or beans for plant-based protein, fiber, and a variety of vitamins and minerals.

## Whole Grains:

**Quinoa Salad:**Create a quinoa salad with colorful vegetables like tomatoes, cucumbers, and bell peppers for a nutrient-packed side.

**Sweet Potatoes:**Incorporate sweet potatoes for complex carbohydrates, fiber, and beta-carotene, supporting eye health.

**Vegetables**:

**Spinach and Mushroom Saute:**Prepare a saute of spinach and mushrooms, rich in antioxidants, vitamins, and minerals.

**Steamed Broccoli:**Steam broccoli to retain its nutritional value, providing fiber, vitamin C, and folate.

**Healthy Fats:**

**Salmon Fillet:**Enjoy a grilled or baked salmon fillet for omega-3 fatty acids, beneficial for heart health and cognitive function.

**Mixed Nuts:**Include a handful of mixed nuts for a dose of healthy fats, antioxidants, and minerals.

**Dairy or Dairy Alternatives:**

**Greek Yogurt with Berries:**Opt for Greek yogurt with fresh berries for a calcium-rich and probiotic-packed dessert.

**Almond Milk:**Choose almond milk as a dairy alternative, fortified with vitamins D and E.

**Hydration**:

**Herbal Tea:**Conclude the meal with a cup of herbal tea for hydration and potential digestive benefits.

**Spices and Herbs:**

**Turmeric and Ginger:**Incorporate turmeric and ginger into dishes for their anti-inflammatory properties.

**Portion Control:**

**Balanced Portions:**Be mindful of portion sizes to maintain a healthy weight and avoid overeating.

**Limit Processed Foods and Sodium:**

**Homemade Dressings:**Make homemade dressings to control sodium intake and enhance the flavor of salads.

**Customization and Adaptation:**

**Personal Preferences:**Customize the dinner based on personal taste preferences while still focusing on nutrient-rich options.

**Regular Check-ins:**Regularly assess dietary needs and make adjustments as necessary, considering any changes in health or lifestyle.

This well-rounded dinner plan emphasizes nutrient density, a variety of food groups, and addresses specific nutritional needs for men above 60, promoting overall health and well-being.

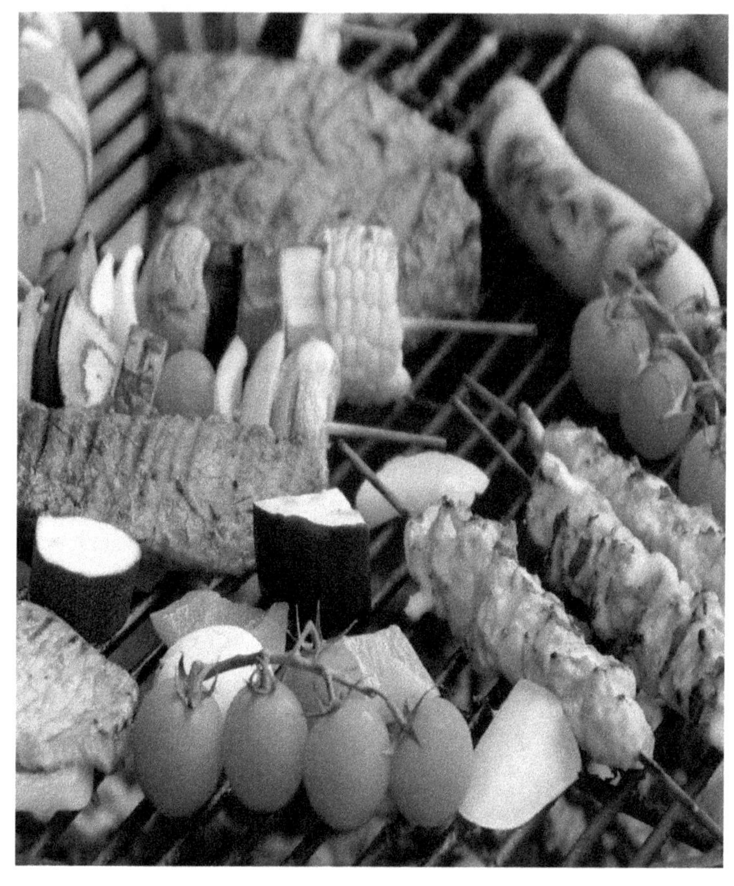

# CHAPTER THREE

## Snack Ideas for Sustained Energy for Men Over 60

As men age, maintaining sustained energy levels becomes crucial for overall well-being. Chapter 6 focuses on providing nutritious snack ideas tailored to meet the specific needs of men over 60. These snacks are designed to support energy levels, promote satiety, and address nutritional requirements associated with aging.

**Nuts and Seeds Mix:**A blend of almonds, walnuts, and pumpkin seeds offers a rich source of omega-3 fatty acids and antioxidants, supporting brain health and combating inflammation.

**Greek Yogurt Parfait:**Combining Greek yogurt with fresh berries and a sprinkle of granola creates a snack rich in protein, probiotics, and fiber, promoting digestive health and muscle maintenance.

**Hummus and Vegetable Sticks:**Hummus, made from chickpeas, provides a protein boost, while colorful vegetable sticks like carrots and bell peppers offer essential vitamins and minerals.

**Whole Grain Crackers with Cheese:**Opt for whole grain crackers paired with a serving of cheese to provide a balanced combination of carbohydrates, protein, and healthy fats for

sustained energy.

**Trail Mix with Dried Fruits:**A mix of nuts,

seeds, and dried fruits provides a portable and

energy-dense snack, offering a quick source of

natural sugars and nutrients.

**Hard-Boiled Eggs:**Eggs are an excellent

source of many different nutrients and protein.

Hard-boiled eggs make for a convenient snack

that supports muscle health and provides

long-lasting energy.

**Smoothie with Protein Powder:**Blend

together a mix of fruits, vegetables, and protein

powder to create a nutrient-packed smoothie

that addresses protein needs and provides a

quick energy boost.

**Avocado Toast on Whole Grain Bread:**Avocado is rich in healthy fats, while whole grain bread offers complex carbohydrates. This combination helps maintain stable blood sugar levels and provides sustained energy.

**Cottage Cheese with Pineapple:**Cottage cheese is a good source of protein, and pairing it with pineapple adds a touch of sweetness along with vitamins and enzymes that aid digestion.

**Sardines on Whole Grain Crackers:**Sardines are an excellent source of protein and are high in omega-3 fatty acids. Combined with whole grain crackers, this snack supports heart health and energy levels.

It's essential for men over 60 to focus on nutrient-dense snacks that contribute to overall health and well-being. These snack ideas aim to provide sustained energy, promote satiety, and address specific nutritional needs associated with aging. As always, individuals should consult with healthcare professionals for personalized dietary advice based on their health status and individual requirements.

## Cooking Techniques for Retaining Nutrients

Preserving nutrients during cooking is crucial for maintaining the nutritional value of your meals. Here are some cooking techniques that help retain essential nutrients in your food:

**Steam Cooking:**A mild cooking technique that reduces nutrient loss is steaming. It involves using hot steam to cook food, keeping vitamins and minerals intact.

This technique is particularly effective for vegetables, as it helps maintain their vibrant colors and prevents the leaching of water-soluble nutrients.

**Microwaving:**Microwaving is a quick and efficient method that generally retains more nutrients than traditional cooking methods.

It cooks food by producing heat directly within the food, reducing the exposure to prolonged high temperatures that can degrade nutrients.

**Sautéing and Stir-Frying:**These methods involve cooking food quickly over high heat with minimal water. This helps in preserving water-soluble vitamins like vitamin C and some B vitamins.Use small amounts of healthy oils, such as olive oil, to enhance the absorption of fat-soluble vitamins like A, D, E, and K.

**Blanching:**Blanching involves briefly immersing vegetables in boiling water, followed by rapid cooling in ice water. This method helps to retain color, texture, and nutrients.It's an effective technique for vegetables like broccoli and spinach.

**Grilling and Roasting:**While high-temperature cooking methods like grilling and roasting can lead to some nutrient loss, they can also enhance the flavors of certain foods.To minimize nutrient degradation, marinate meats with herbs and spices, which can provide antioxidants that counteract potential damage.

**Pressure Cooking:**Pressure cooking uses steam and high pressure to cook food quickly. This method helps in preserving water-soluble vitamins and minerals.It's particularly beneficial for legumes and whole grains, reducing cooking time and nutrient loss.

**Use Cooking Water:**When boiling vegetables, consider using the cooking water in soups or stews to retain some of the nutrients that leach into the water.

**Avoid Overcooking:**Overcooking can lead to nutrient degradation. Cook foods until they are just tender to avoid unnecessary nutrient loss.

**Use Fresh Ingredients:**The quality of your ingredients matters. Fresh produce tends to have higher nutrient content than older, wilted counterparts.

**Store and Reheat Properly:**Proper storage and reheating techniques help in maintaining nutrient levels. Store leftovers promptly in the refrigerator and reheat them using methods that don't further degrade nutrients.

Incorporating these cooking techniques into your culinary practices can help you prepare delicious and nutritious meals that contribute to overall health and well-being.

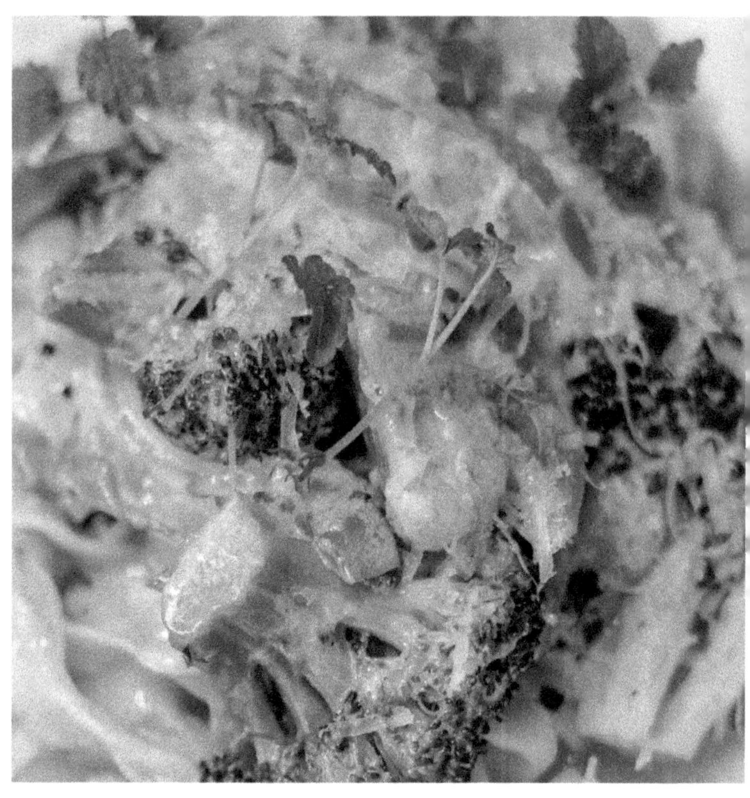

# CHAPTER FOUR

**Easy-to-Follow Recipes for men above 60;**Certainly! Here's a set of easy-to-follow recipes tailored for men above 60, taking into consideration their nutritional **needs and preferences:**

1. **Oatmeal with Berries and Nuts:**

**Ingredients**:Old-fashioned oats,Mixed berries (blueberries, strawberries),Chopped nuts (walnuts, almonds),Milk or yogurt

**Instructions**:Cook oats according to package instructions.Top with a handful of mixed berries and a sprinkle of chopped nuts.Add milk or yogurt for creaminess.

## 2. **Vegetable Omelette:**

**Ingredients**:Eggs,Chopped bell peppers, tomatoes, and spinach,Cheese (optional),Salt and pepper

**Instructions**;Whisk eggs and pour into a heated, non-stick pan.Add chopped veggies and cook until eggs set.Add cheese if desired and fold the omelette.

## 3. **Salmon Salad:**

**Ingredients**:Grilled or baked salmon.Mixed salad greens.Cherry tomatoes.Olive oil and balsamic vinegar dressing.

**Instructions**:Flake the salmon over a bed of mixed greens and tomatoes.Drizzle with balsamic vinegar dressing and olive oil.

## 4. Slow Cooker Chicken Stew:

**Ingredients**:Chicken thighs,Potatoes, carrots, celery,Chicken broth,Herbs and spices

**Instructions**:Place chicken and chopped vegetables in a slow cooker.Add chicken broth, herbs, and spices.Cook on low for 6-8 hours until everything is tender.

## 5. **Quinoa Stir-Fry:**

**Ingredients**:Quinoa,Various stir-fried veggies, including snap peas, bell peppers, and broccol,iSoy sauce,Sesame oil.

**Instructions**:Cook quinoa according to package instructions.Stir-fry vegetables in sesame oil and add cooked quinoa.Drizzle with soy sauce and toss until well combined.

## 6. **Greek Yogurt Parfait:**

**Ingredients**:Greek yogurt,Honey,Mixed nuts and granola,Fresh fruits (berries, banana slices)

**Instructions**:Layer Greek yogurt, honey, nuts, granola, and fresh fruits.Repeat for a delicious and nutritious parfait.

These recipes focus on incorporating essential nutrients, fiber, and protein while keeping the preparation simple and flavorful. Adjust portion sizes based on individual preferences and dietary needs.

# Types of soup and stew for men above 60, include ingredients and how to prepare them

Certainly! Here are two hearty and nutritious soup and stew options that are well-suited for men above 60:

## Chicken and Vegetable Soup

Ingredients:

- 1 whole chicken, cut into pieces
- 2 carrots, peeled and sliced
- 2 celery stalks, chopped
- 1 onion, diced
- 3 cloves garlic, minced

- 1 cup green beans, chopped

- 1 cup corn kernels

- 1 cup peas

- 8 cups chicken broth

- 1 teaspoon dried thyme

- 1 bay leaf

- Salt and pepper to taste

- Fresh parsley for garnish

**Instructions**:

- In a large pot, bring the chicken broth to a boil.

- Add the chicken pieces, carrots, celery, onion, and garlic to the pot.

- Season with dried thyme, bay leaf, salt, and pepper.

- Reduce the heat to a simmer and let it cook for about 30-40 minutes until the chicken is fully cooked.
- Remove the chicken from the pot, shred the meat, and return it to the soup.
- Add green beans, corn, and peas. Simmer for an additional 10-15 minutes.
- Adjust seasoning as needed.
- Garnish with fresh parsley before serving.

**Beef and Barley Stew**

**Ingredients**:

- 1.5 lbs stewing beef, cubed
- 1 cup barley
- 2 carrots, peeled and sliced

- 2 potatoes, diced

- 1 onion, finely chopped

- 3 cloves garlic, minced

- 4 cups beef broth

- 1 cup red wine (optional)

- 1 tablespoon tomato paste

- 1 teaspoon dried thyme

- Salt and pepper to taste

- Olive oil for cooking

**Instructions:**

- Warm up the olive oil in a big pot over medium-high heat.

- Brown the beef cubes on all sides after adding them.

- Add the minced garlic and onion, and cook until they become tender.

- Add the tomato paste and let it cook for a few minutes.

- Deglaze the pot by adding the red wine, if using  to deglaze the pot. to deglaze the pot.

- Add carrots, potatoes, and barley to the pot.

- Pour in the beef broth, add dried thyme, salt, and pepper.

- Bring to a boil, then reduce heat and simmer for 1.5 to 2 hours until beef is tender and flavors meld.

- Adjust seasoning as needed before serving.

Both of these recipes provide a good balance of protein, vegetables, and carbohydrates, making them suitable for the dietary needs of men above 60. Additionally, they can be easily customized based on personal preferences and nutritional requirements.

# Grilled and Baked Dishes for men above 60 also include ingredients and how to prepare them

Certainly! Here's a compilation of grilled and baked dishes suitable for men above 60, along with their ingredients and preparation instructions:

1. **Grilled Salmon with Lemon Herb Marinade:**
   - Ingredients:
     1. Salmon fillets
     2. Lemon juice

3. Olive oil

4. Fresh herbs (such as dill, parsley, and thyme)

5. Garlic cloves

6. Salt and pepper to taste

- Preparation:

1. Combine lemon juice, olive oil, minced garlic, chopped herbs, salt, and pepper to create the marinade.

2. Marinate salmon fillets for at least 30 minutes.

3. Grill the salmon until it flakes easily with a fork.

## 2. Baked Chicken Breast with Rosemary and Garlic:

- Ingredients:

1. Chicken breasts

2. Olive oil

3. Fresh rosemary

4. Garlic cloves

5. Paprika

6. Salt and pepper to taste

- Preparation:

   1. Preheat the oven and brush chicken breasts with olive oil.

   2. Season with chopped rosemary, minced garlic, paprika, salt, and pepper.

   3. Bake until the chicken is cooked through.

3. **Grilled Vegetable Skewers:**

- Ingredients:

   1. Bell peppers (assorted colors)

   2. Zucchini

   3. Cherry tomatoes

4. Red onion

5. Olive oil

6. Balsamic vinegar

7. Italian seasoning

8. Salt and pepper to taste

- Preparation:

  1. Cut vegetables into bite-sized pieces.

  2. Thread onto skewers and brush with a mixture of olive oil, balsamic vinegar, Italian seasoning, salt, and pepper.

  3. Grill until vegetables are tender.

## 4. Baked Cod with Lemon Butter Sauce:

- Ingredients:

  1. Cod fillets

2. Lemon zest and juice

3. Butter

4. Garlic powder

5. Dill

6. Salt and pepper to taste

- Preparation:

1. Place cod fillets in a baking dish.

2. Mix melted butter, lemon zest, lemon juice, garlic powder, dill, salt, and pepper.

3. Pour the sauce over the cod and bake until fish flakes easily.

5. **Grilled Pork Chops with Apple Cider Glaze:**

- Ingredients:

1. Pork chops

2. Apple cider

        3. Dijon mustard

        4. Brown sugar

        5. Thyme

        6. Salt and pepper to taste

    ○ Preparation:

        1. Season pork chops with salt and pepper.

        2. Grill until cooked through.

        3. Combine apple cider, Dijon mustard, brown sugar, and thyme in a saucepan. Simmer until it thickens into a glaze.

These dishes provide a mix of lean proteins and colorful vegetables, rich in flavor and nutrients. Adjust seasonings according to personal taste preferences. Always consider any dietary restrictions or preferences when preparing meals.

# Vegetarian Options for men above 60 also include recipes, ingredients and how to prepare them

Certainly! A vegetarian diet for men above 60 can be rich in nutrients that support overall health. Here are some nutritious vegetarian options along with recipes, ingredients, and preparation instructions:

1. **Quinoa Salad:**

Ingredients:

- Quinoa

- Mixed vegetables (bell peppers, cucumber, cherry tomatoes)

- Feta cheese

- Olive oil

- Lemon juice

- Fresh herbs (parsley, mint)

Preparation:

- Cook quinoa according to package instructions.

- Chop vegetables and mix with cooked quinoa.

- Crumble feta cheese on top.

- Dress with olive oil, lemon juice, and fresh herbs.

2. **Lentil Soup:**

Ingredients:

- Green or brown lentils

- Carrots, onions, celery

- Garlic

- Vegetable broth

- Cumin, coriander, thyme

- Spinach or kale

Preparation:

- Sauté onions, carrots, celery, and garlic.

- Add lentils, vegetable broth, and spices.

- Simmer until lentils are tender.

- Stir in greens before serving.

3. **Stir-Fried Tofu with Vegetables:**

Ingredients:

- Firm tofu

- Broccoli, bell peppers, snap peas

- Soy sauce, ginger, garlic

- Sesame oil

Preparation:

- Press and cube tofu; stir-fry until golden.
- Add chopped vegetables and sauté.
- Mix soy sauce, ginger, and garlic; pour over tofu and veggies.
- Drizzle with sesame oil before serving.

## 4. **Sweet Potato and Chickpea Curry:**

Ingredients:

- Sweet potatoes, chickpeas
- Onion, tomatoes, garlic, ginger
- Coconut milk
- Curry spices (turmeric, cumin, coriander)

Preparation:

- Sauté onions, garlic, and ginger.

- Add sweet potatoes, chickpeas, tomatoes, and spices.

- Pour in coconut milk; simmer until potatoes are tender.

## 5. **Mushroom and Spinach Stuffed Bell Peppers**:

Ingredients:

- Bell peppers

- Mushrooms, spinach, onions, garlic

- Brown rice

- Tomato sauce

- Italian seasoning

Preparation:

- Cook brown rice; sauté mushrooms, onions, and garlic.

- Mix in spinach, rice, and Italian seasoning.
- Stuff peppers, top with tomato sauce, and bake.

## 6. Greek Yogurt Parfait:

Ingredients:

- Greek yogurt
- Mixed berries
- Granola
- Honey

Preparation:

- Layer Greek yogurt, berries, and granola.
- Drizzle with honey before serving.

These recipes provide a variety of nutrients crucial for maintaining health in men above 60, including fiber, protein, vitamins, and minerals.

Depending on dietary requirements and personal preferences, modify ingredient and quantity sizes. For individualized guidance, always seek the assistance of a healthcare practitioner.

# Healthy Desserts for men above 60 also include recipes, ingredients and preparations

Certainly! Healthy desserts for men above 60 can be both delicious and nutritious. Here are some ideas along with recipes, ingredients;

## 1. **Baked Apple with Cinnamon:**

Ingredients:

- 2 medium-sized apples
- 1 teaspoon cinnamon
- 1 tablespoon honey

Preparation:

- Preheat the oven to 375°F (190°C).
- After coreing the apples, transfer them to a baking dish.
- Mix cinnamon with honey and drizzle over the apples.
- Bake for 25-30 minutes or until the apples are tender.

## 2. **Greek Yogurt Parfait:**

Ingredients:

- 1 cup Greek yogurt

- 1/2 cup mixed berries (blueberries, strawberries)

- 2 tablespoons granola

- 1 tablespoon honey

Preparation:

- Arrange granola, mixed berries, and Greek yogurt in a glass.
- Drizzle honey on top for sweetness.

3. **Chia Seed Pudding:**

Ingredients:

- 3 tablespoons chia seeds

- 1 cup almond milk

- 1/2 teaspoon vanilla extract

- 1 tablespoon maple syrup

Preparation:

- In a bowl, combine chia seeds, almond milk, maple syrup, and vanilla essence.

- Refrigerate for at least 4 hours or overnight until it thickens.

- 4. Frozen Banana Bites:

Ingredients:

- 2 ripe bananas

- 1/4 cup dark chocolate, melted

- 1/4 cup chopped nuts (almonds, walnuts)

Preparation:

- Slice bananas into rounds.

- Dip each banana slice in melted chocolate, then coat with chopped nuts.

- Freeze for 2 hours.

5. **Avocado Chocolate Mousse:**

Ingredients:

- 2 ripe avocados
- 1/4 cup cocoa powder
- 1/4 cup honey
- 1 teaspoon vanilla extract

Preparation:

- Smoothly blend avocados, cocoa powder, honey, and vanilla.
- Refrigerate before serving.

## 6. Oatmeal Raisin Cookies:

Ingredients:

- 1 cup oats
- 1/2 cup whole wheat flour
- 1/2 cup raisins
- 1/4 cup coconut oil
- 1/4 cup maple syrup

Preparation:

- Mix oats, whole wheat flour, raisins, melted coconut oil, and maple syrup.
- Shape into cookies and bake at 350°F (175°C) for 12-15 minutes.

These desserts are rich in nutrients, low in added sugars, and provide essential vitamins and antioxidants suitable for men above 60. Always get the advice of a medical expert before making any dietary changes. Enjoy these guilt-free treats!

# CHAPTER FIVE

## The types of Exercise and Nutrition Synergy for men above 60

Exercise and nutrition synergy is crucial for promoting overall health and well-being in men above 60. As individuals age, maintaining a balance between physical activity and proper nutrition becomes increasingly important. Here are various types of exercises and nutritional considerations that synergistically contribute to the well-being of older men:

**Types of Exercise:**

**Cardiovascular Exercise:**

Activities like brisk walking, cycling, or swimming help improve heart health and maintain cardiovascular fitness.

Aim for at least 150 minutes of aerobic activity per week, which can be 75 minutes of vigorous exercise or moderate to severe exercise.

Focus on resistance exercises to maintain muscle mass and strength.

Include weightlifting, resistance band workouts, or bodyweight exercises in the routine.

Strength training can improve bone density and reduce the risk of falls.

**Flexibility and Balance Training:**

Incorporate stretching exercises to enhance flexibility and maintain a full range of motion.

Balance exercises, such as yoga or tai chi, are beneficial for preventing falls and improving overall stability.

**Low-Impact Activities:**

Consider activities with minimal joint impact, like elliptical training or water aerobics, to protect joints while staying active.

**Nutrition Considerations:**

Protein Intake:

Adequate protein consumption is crucial for maintaining muscle mass and promoting muscle repair.

Include lean protein sources like fish, poultry, beans, and low-fat dairy in meals.

**Calcium and Vitamin D:**

Support bone health by ensuring sufficient calcium intake, either through dietary sources or supplements.

Combine this with vitamin D to enhance calcium absorption, promoting bone density.

**Hydration:**

Older individuals may have a reduced sense of thirst, making dehydration a concern. Water should be consumed in moderation throughout the day.

Include hydrating foods like fruits and vegetables in the diet.

**Fiber-Rich Foods:**

Incorporate fiber to support digestive health and maintain a healthy weight.

Fruits, vegetables, and whole grains are all great sources of dietary fiber.

**Balanced Diet:**

Aim for a well-rounded diet that includes a variety of nutrients. Pay close attention to fruits, vegetables, whole grains, lean meats, and healthy fats.

Consider consulting a nutritionist to tailor dietary recommendations to individual needs.

Synergy:

**Preventing Muscle Loss:**

Combining strength training with sufficient protein intake helps counteract age-related muscle loss.

**Joint Health:**

Low-impact exercises, coupled with anti-inflammatory foods, contribute to joint health and reduce the risk of arthritis-related issues.

**Overall Well-Being:**

The combination of regular exercise and a balanced diet contributes to improved mood, cognitive function, and overall quality of life.

**Weight Management:**

Synergistic efforts in both nutrition and exercise help manage weight, reducing the risk of obesity-related conditions.

In conclusion, the synergy between exercise and nutrition is pivotal for promoting health and vitality in men above 60. Tailoring these components to individual needs, considering existing health conditions, and seeking professional guidance contribute to a holistic approach to aging gracefully.

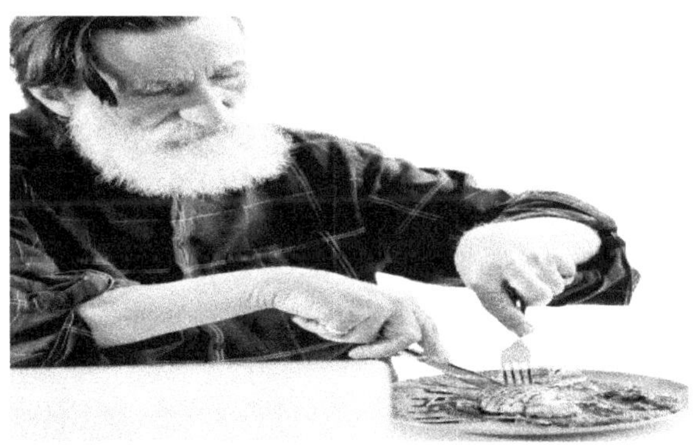

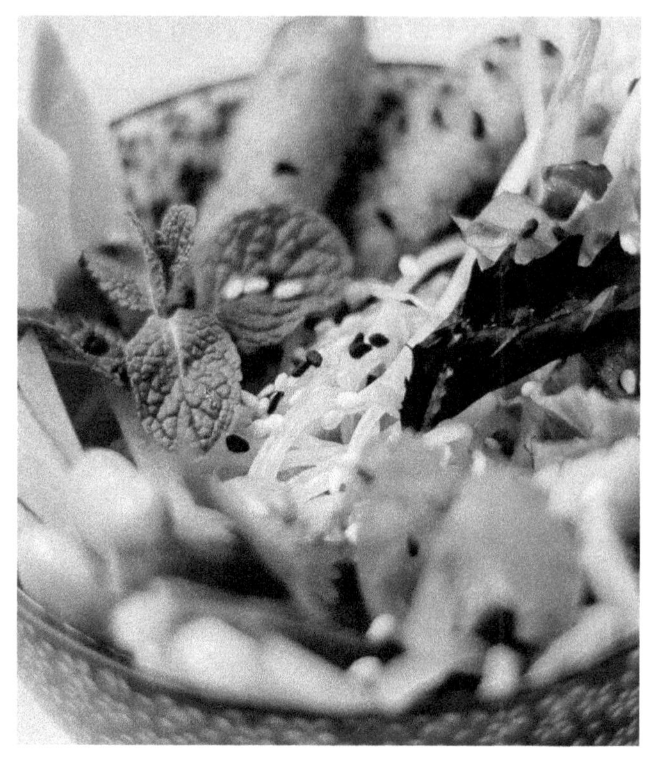

# CHAPTER SIX

## Embracing a Healthy Lifestyle for men above 60

Embracing a healthy lifestyle is crucial for men above 60 to maintain overall well-being and enhance the quality of life. This involves incorporating a balanced diet, regular physical activity, adequate sleep, stress management, and regular health check-ups into their daily routine.

1. **Balanced Diet:**

Make eating a diet rich in fruits, vegetables, lean meats, complete grains, and healthy fats a priority

Include foods high in calcium and vitamin D for bone health, such as dairy products, leafy greens, and fortified foods.

Limit processed foods, sugary snacks, and excessive salt intake to prevent conditions like hypertension and diabetes.

## 2. Regular Exercise:

Engage in a combination of aerobic exercises (walking, swimming) and strength training to maintain cardiovascular health and muscle mass.

## 3. Adequate Sleep:

Ensure 7-9 hours of sleep per night to support physical and mental well-being.

Create a cozy sleeping environment and stick to a regular sleep schedule.

## 4. Stress Management:

Practice stress-reducing techniques like meditation, deep breathing, or yoga to alleviate mental and emotional strain.

Take part in enjoyable and relaxing hobbies and activities.

## 5. Regular Health Check-ups:

Schedule regular check-ups with healthcare professionals to monitor blood pressure, cholesterol levels, and other vital markers.

Screenings for conditions like prostate cancer and colon cancer become more important with age.

# Examples of a Day in a Healthy Lifestyle for Men Above 60:

**Breakfast:**

- Oatmeal with berries and a handful of nuts.
- Low-fat yogurt or a smoothie with spinach and banana.
- Mid-Morning Snack:
- Fresh fruit like an apple or a handful of almonds.

**Lunch:**

- Grilled chicken or fish with a variety of colorful vegetables.
- Quinoa or brown rice as a side.

**Afternoon Snack:**

- Greek yogurt or a small serving of cottage cheese.

**Dinner**:

- Baked salmon with steamed broccoli and sweet potatoes.
- A mixed salad with dark leafy greens.

**Evening**:

- A brisk 30-minute walk or light stretching exercises.

**Before Bed:**

- Herbal tea or warm milk to promote relaxation.

Remember, consulting with healthcare professionals before making significant lifestyle changes is advisable. Tailoring these recommendations to individual health

conditions and preferences is crucial for

long-term success in adopting a healthy

lifestyle for men above 60.

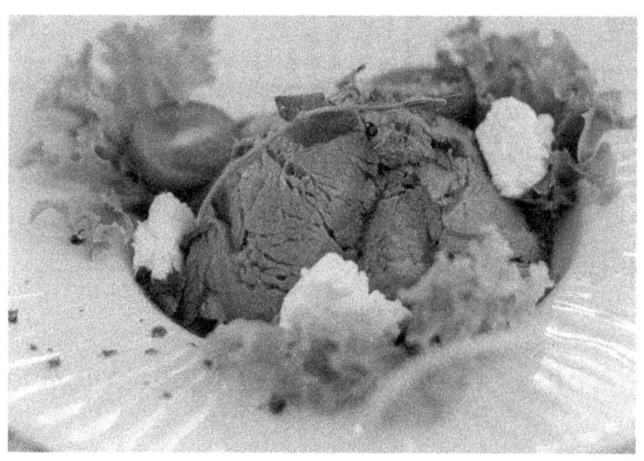

# Conclusion

In conclusion, a healthy eating cookbook tailored for men above 60 is not only a practical guide to culinary choices but a testament to the importance of nutrition in promoting overall well-being during this stage of life. The recipes within this cookbook  focuses on nutrient-dense, balanced meals that cater to the specific nutritional needs of aging men, encompassing a variety of vitamins, minerals, and essential nutrients.

This cookbook serves as a valuable resource, offering not just a collection of recipes but a comprehensive approach to maintaining optimal health in later years. It addresses common health concerns such as heart health, bone density, and cognitive function by incorporating ingredients rich in omega-3 fatty acids, calcium, and antioxidants. Moreover, the inclusion of recipes that consider dietary restrictions, ensures that the cookbook is accessible and beneficial to a wide range of individuals.

Beyond the immediate health benefits, this cookbook encourages a positive shift in lifestyle, fostering a greater appreciation for the connection between nutrition and longevity. It empowers men above 60 to take charge of their health through mindful food choices, establishing habits that can contribute to a higher quality of life.

In essence, Healthy Eating Cookbook for Men Above 60 is more than a culinary guide – it is a holistic approach to aging gracefully through nourishing the body and mind. By embracing the principles laid out in this cookbook, individuals can embark on a journey towards enhanced vitality, improved resilience, and a more fulfilling life in their senior years.

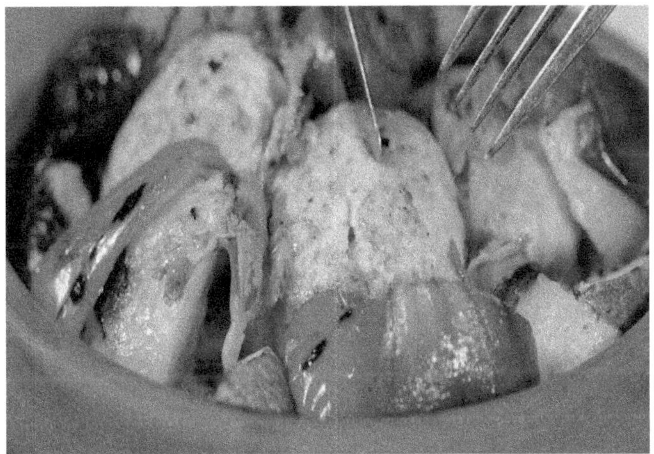

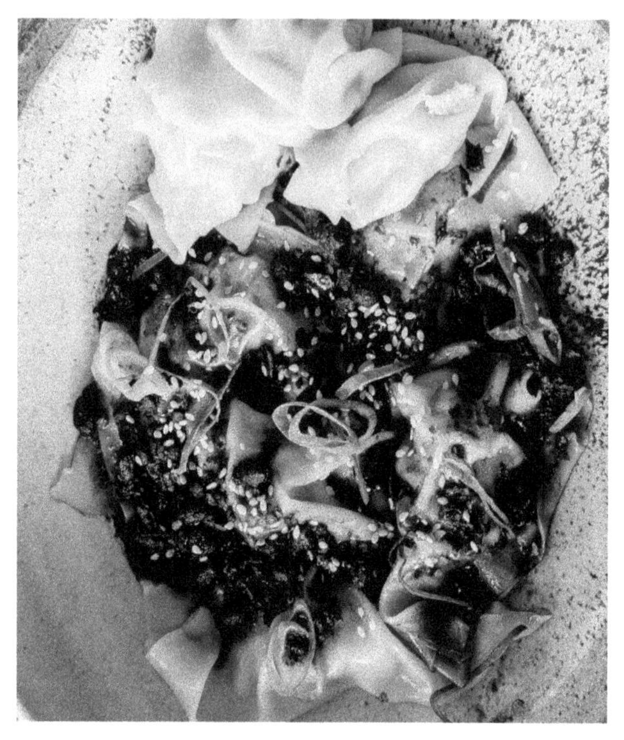

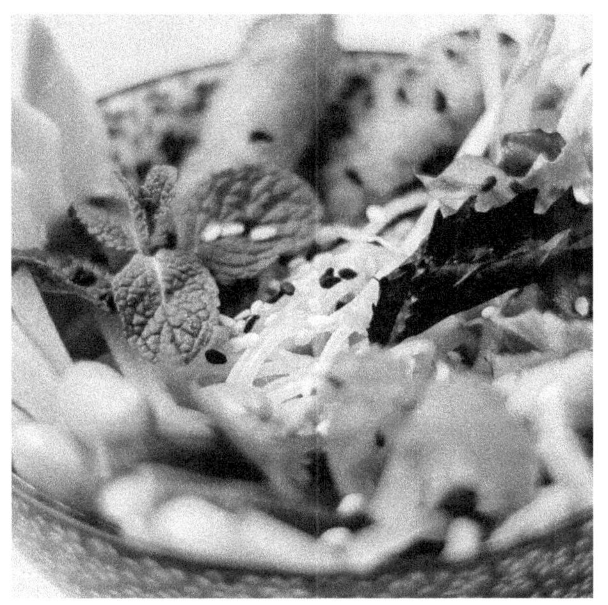